Kinktionary

By 

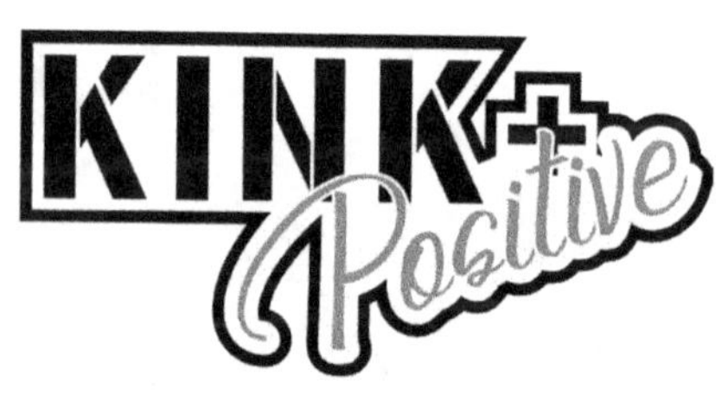

Dedicated

...to those who came before us and helped pull kink out of the shadows, making it more accessible for generations to come.

...to those who continue to forge new kink education pathways that grow with our understanding of kink, sexuality, and the world around us.

...to those who will pick up and continue to carry the kink educational torch in the future.

Contents

Preface

While the world of kink and BDSM is far from new, the language we use to discuss it is constantly evolving and growing while we gain a better understanding of ourselves and the world around us.

What was once a binary system with assumed roles based on gender, we now have fluidity and questions before assumption, or at least we're doing what we can to help that shift so that all consenting adults are included rather than shamed or outcast because they don't fit the mold.

This dictionary, the "Kinktionary," is created with this positive growth in mind. A dictionary that updates our old definitions while also providing space for new words and phrases as you come across them. Every section has designated space so you can continue to update definitions as they change, add new words that may be added to our lexicon, and watch your dictionary grow along with you.

Newbies fear not, with over 400 words and phrases contained in "Kinktionary" you're sure to start with a solid foundation for your kink journey. Already an experienced kinkster? Keep "Kinktionary" on hand for quick reference material and add to it to your heart's content.

So, get out your favorite pens, start clipping images of your favorite gear or inspiration for play you love, this isn't your standard school dictionary; in this book you're encouraged to write, draw, scribble, and make it your own!

Abbreviations & Acronyms

24/7	Twentyfour-seven. Shorthand to signifify that someone is involved in the lifestyle all day, every day; it is part of who they are.
B/D or BD	Bondage and Discipline.
BBC	Big black cock.
BBW	Big beautiful women.
BBP	Bloodborne pathogens.
BDSM	Bondage, Discipline, Dominance, Submission, Sadism, and Masochism.
BIPOC	Black, indigenous, and people of color.
CBT	Cock and ball torture.
CNC	Consensual non-consent.
D/s	Dominance/submission or Dominant/submissive.

FF	Face fucking.
LTR	Long term relationship.
M/s	Master/slave.
NRE	New relationship energy.
O/p	Owner/property.
OTK	Over the knee.
PRICK	Personal responsibility in consensual kink.
RACK	Risk aware consensual kink.
RASH	Risk aware, shit happens.
S/M or SM	Sadism and masochism.
SAM	Smart ass masochist.
SSC	Safe, sane, and consensual.
STD/STI	Sexually transmitted disesase/infection.

TT	Tit torture.
WIITWD	What it is that we do.
WS	Watersports.
YKINMK	Your kink is not my kink
YKINMKATO	Your kink is not my kink and that's ok
YKINMKBYKIOK	Your kink is not my kink but your kink is ok

Heard of any others that weren't covered?

Add them below and update your list as new additions are created.

__________ ______________________

____

__________ ______________________

____

__________ ______________________

Words & Phrases

Abduction Play	Play that is centered around the fantasy of being taken by force, kidnapped.
Abrasion Play	Use of materials that scratch, scrape, and rub the surface of the skin.
Age Play	Umbrella term for forms of play that involve playing with age regression or role play, such as littles and adult babies. Participants are adults, children are never involved.
Agender	Term used for someone who doesn't identify as having any gender.
Anal	Shorthand for Anal Sex; sex involving penetrating the anus.

Anal Fisting	The practice of inserting one's fist into someone's anus.
Anal Hook	A large hook shaped sex toy that usually has a ball on the insertion end and a loop at the other end so it can be tied off to something. (See figure on pg 125)
Androgyny	When someone has gender expression characteristics that are both male and female in appearance resulting in expression that is more ambiguous.
Anticipatory Service	Service provided by the submissive in a D/s dynamic that isn't specifically asked for but instead is decided on

_______________________   _______________________

____

_______________________   _______________________

based on context clues and assumptions from previous encounters. ie: refilling an empty cup without being asked

Apprentice Someone who has taken on learning kink skills from a more experienced practitioner.

Armbinder A piece of gear, usually leather, that is used to bind the arms together in one sleeve behind the back. (See figure on pg 125)

Aromantic Someone who has no romantic attraction to other people.

Asexual Someone who has no sexual attraction to other people.

Asphyxiophilia Fetish for being strangled or

unable to breathe.

Ass Play   Any play that involves the anus: anal sex, fisting, plugs, and so on.

Ass to Mouth   Oral sex involving the anus.

Auralism   Sexual arousal to sounds.

Autagonistophilia

Fetish for being on stage, on display, or on camera.

Autassassinophilia

A fetish for being in life-threatening situations.

Auto-Eroticism   To get sexually aroused or satisfied by yourself, without external stimulus.

Ball Gag	A type of gag that has a ball that goes into the mouth to keep the mouth open and prevent anything from going in. (See figure on pg 126)
Ball Stretching	Play that involves stretching the scrotal sack, often through use of weights or wide materials wrapped around the scrotum.
Balloon	Someone who has a fetish for balloons. This can include the balloons in their filled state and/or popping balloons.
Big	Someone involved in Age Play who identifies on the older side of the age spectrum, such as mommies, daddies, and babysitters.

__________ _______________________

____

__________ _______________________

____

Bimbofication   Play that involves transforming
a subject into a bimbo, an
attractive and flighty female
character.

Biromantic   Once thought to be romantic
attraction to both male and
female partners but now
is used to say a romantic
attraction to one's own gender
and others.

Bisexual   Once thought to be sexual
attraction to both male and
female partners but now is
used to say a sexual attraction
to one's own gender and
others.

Blindfold   A piece of gear that is used
to cover the eyes. Can be
made out of a wide variety

_______________   _______________________

                   ____

_______________   _______________________

of materials including being
improvised with common
household items.
(See figure on pg 126)

Blood Choke A form of breath play that
involves restricting blood flow
to control oxygen movement
rather than inhibiting one's
ability to breathe.

Blood Play Play that centers around
playing with blood; not the
same as vampirism.

**Body
Modification** A wide range of alterations
that can be done to the body
such as piercings, tattoos,
brands, scarring, and plastic
surgery.

Body Worship   Adoration for specific parts of or the whole body.

Boi   Alternative spelling for "boy" typically used by people who present masculine but do not identify as male.

Bondage   Umbrella term for all forms of physical restraining methods. Includes play like rope, mummification, cuffs, cages, and straps.

Bondage Tape   Self adhering plastic tape that contains no adhesives or glues and comes in a wide range of colors.

Boot Worship   Devotion and praise directed towards boots that the participant finds desirable.

_______________   _______________

_______________   _______________

_______________   _______________

Bootblack	Someone who cares for boots and other leather items through cleaning, conditioning, polishing, and refinishing.
Bootblacking	The process of caring for boots and leather items through cleaning, conditioning, polishing, and refinishing.
Bottom	To be on the receiving end of an activity; bottoming is not the same as submitting. For example: to bottom for flogging means you are getting flogged, to bottom for a massage means you are being massaged.
Boundaries	Dividing lines between what is and isn't acceptable in play, relationships, or any other

____

____

____

negotiated situation.

Boy
A title used mainly by submissive men in kink communities; counter to "Sir" which is typically for dominant men.

Branding
Use of heat or cold to leave a scar/mark on the skin.

Brat
Label used to signify a submissive who enjoys misbehaving and being mischievous with their partner.

Breast Bondage
Binding of the chest specifically to accentuate and draw attention to the breasts. While commonly done on women, people of all gender

can engage in this activity.

Breath Play/Control	Play that involves restricting and controlling oxygen intake.
Bukkake	The act of having multiple men ejaculate onto someone's face.
Bullwhip	A singletail whip that is usually made up of braided leather or nylon cording. Originally used for livestock herding through the use of loud cracking sounds. (See figure on pg 131)
Butch	Having the characteristics of being masculine in appearance and mannerisms.

Butler Book	A book or journal used to keep track of household information from resident biographical info to utility billing info and more.
Butt Plug	A flanged sex toy that looks similar to a dildo but is designed to be worn inside the anus for an extended period. (See figure on pg 125)
Cage	A structure made up of bars, wires, cables, or similar slatted material designed to confine a person or specific body parts. (See figure on pg 129)
Canes	Thin and slightly flexible rods that are used for impact play. Can be made from natural materials like bamboo or synthetic ones like fiberglass.

	(See figure on pg 130)
Caning	Impact play done specifically with a cane, not a walking stick. Can be mild with light tapping and build from there.
Capnolagnia	To be aroused by smoking.
Captivity	To be confined or imprisoned in a cage or other form of bondage.
Caregiver	Role where someone is in charge of the care of another person, such as a little or ward. Caregiver/Little may be used as an alternative to Daddy or Mommy and Little.
Cat O'Nine Tails	Flogger like implement made

with exactly nine tails/falls
that are usually braided and
attached to a handle.
(See figure on pg 130)

Catharsis

A state of highly emotional
release of tension that
typically follows an intense
scene and often paired with
"ugly crying."

Catheterization

Play that involves putting a
catheter into the urinary tract,
sometimes for the purpose of
collecting urine in a collection
bag.

Cell Popping

Use of heated metal or violet
wand to create microbranding
on the skin.

Chaps

Leather pants that are made

without the crotch or seat. "Assless chaps" is a redundant statement as all chaps are assless.

Chastity

To refrain from sexual activity. In kink settings this is often done via chastity devices that lock off access to the genitals.

Chastity Belt

A belt that locks on to the body to prevent access to one's sexual organs.

Chastity Cage

A device designed to lock on to a penis that prevents erection and the ability to masturbate.
(See figure on pg 127)

Check In

Used during a scene to ensure that all parties are happy with what is happening and wish for the play to continue.

Chosen Family A group of people who are not related by blood or birth but instead by choice.

Cigar Play Play that involves cigars, often providing cutting and lighting services, or acting as a human ashtray.

Clamps A piece of gear used to press body parts together or put a single one under pressure from two sides. Some are adjustable and lockable.

Clothespins An item used to hang clothing but acts as a pinching mechanism in kink settings. (See figure on pg 133)

_______________ ___________________________

_______________ ___________________________

_______________ ___________________________

Collar	Similar to those worn by dogs and cats, collars are used to show ownership or status as a submissive in BDSM. Alternative representations include necklaces, bracelets, anklets, and other types of jewelry, or even tattoos. (See figure on pg 126)
Collar and Leash	Similar to a collar and leash used for a dog, these items are used in kink to connect a dominant and submissive partner. In some groups a leash attached to a collar means that the submissive partner is under extra restrictions on who they can and cannot speak to.

Collared

Often viewed as equivalent or similar to being married, or an even deeper connection. Some use multiple collars to signify play partners, committed relationships, training/ engagement, and collared/ married.

Coming Out

The act of disclosing part of one's identity to others such as sexual orientation, gender identity, or kink affiliation.

Conditioning

Training someone to act and respond a certain way to different stimuli.

Condom

Contraceptive barrier used in sex to prevent pregnancy and transmission of STI's.

____

____

____

| **Confinement** | Use of binding methods to restrict movement and create a sense of imprisonment. |

Consensual Non-Consent

Play or relationship status that involves agreeing to a certain set of rules ahead of time which may include things that may push their comfort levels later on. For example: agreeing that "no" will not hold weight in the future and instead a safeword may be required to halt activities.

Consent

Agreeing to engage in an activity or interaction.

Contract

Non-legally binding paperwork that mimics real life contracts for the purpose of

	outlining relationships, play, apprenticeships, and other engagements.
Control	Having the ability to influence another person, group of people, or events.
Corporal Punishment	The use of physical pain as punishment for undesired behavior, such as spankings.
Corset Training	Use of a corset or similar garment to train one's waist into a smaller size.
Counting Strikes	Play activity where the bottom counts aloud each hit from a specific tool or implement, such as a paddle or whip.
Courting	The active process of getting

to know someone in hopes of creating a formal relationship, also known as dating.

Covered   When someone in the Leather community is awarded a Muir cap for the purpose of deeming them a "Master" in their community, similar to a lifetime achievement award. Sometimes they are given the title "Sir" instead.

Cracker   The very bottom of a singletail whip, like a bullwhip, which is responsible for creating the crack sound when thrown. (See figure on pg 131)

Crops   Similar to a crop but the end has a small piece of material on it, usually in the shape of

____________________   ____________________

____________________   ____________________

____

a rectangle or heart and made
of leather or plastic.
(See figure on pg 130)

Cross-Dressing   When someone wears clothes
usually designated for the
opposite sex.

Crucifixion   To bind someone to a cross
using rope or nails.

Cruising   A method of flirting common in
gay bars that relies on non-
verbal communication.

Cuckold   A man involved in a form of
non-monogamy where the wife
has multiple male partners
but each male partner is
monogamous and faithful to
the wife only.

Cuffs	Bindings for the wrists and ankles, often made from leather.
Cunnilingus	Oral sex performed on vulva.
Cupping	Form of play based on therapeutic use of glass or plastic cups to create suction that pulls the skin up and away from the underlying musculature and fascia.
Cuttings	Use of a scalpel or similar cutting instrument to cut the skin, sometimes in decorative patterns, and cause pain.
Dacryphilia	Fetish for and attraction to people crying.
Daddy	Title given to and used by

people who might identify as
a father figure in Age Play
or simply enjoy being called
"Daddy."

**Damsel in
Distress**

Style of bondage that focuses
on old damsel in distress
aesthetics, such as a woman
hog-tied on railroad tracks.

Deal-Breaker

Similar to a hard limit, a deal
breaker is something that
cannot or will not be tolerated
in play, a relationship, or other
engagement.

Degradation

Type of play that focuses
on wearing someone down
verbally, mentally, or
emotionally.

___________________   ___________________________

                        ____

___________________   ___________________________

Dental Dam	A form of personal protective equipment that is used for oral sex on vulvas to prevent STI transmission.
Dildo	An object made for the purpose of insertion into the body for sexual purposes.
Discipline	The desire to follow rules and the training involved with ensuring that rules and protocols are followed.
Dollification	Play that involves transforming someone into a doll to be dressed up and played with, similar to a life-size Barbie.
Domestic Violence	Nonconsensual aggression and violence that occurs within

the home, between domestic partners. Not all domestic violence is physical, it can be mental and emotional as well. See Resources section if you need help.

Dominance   To have the power and influence over another person, consensually.

Dominant   Person in a power exchange relationship who has been consensually given power and influence over the other partner, the submissive partner.

Dominatrix   A term often used for female professional dominants.

Dragontail   A singletail type impact play

toy made from a long roll
of leather with a handle.
Does not have a cracker like
singletail whips.
(See figure on pg 131)

Earned Leather   In some Leather communities
leather clothing can be
earned as a way of showing
achievements and service to
their communities. Earned
leather pieces may or may
not be given with a small
ceremony marking the
occasion.

Edge Play   Play that is on the "edge" of
safety or is considered very
risky. Some places classify any
play with a sharp edge and
potential for blood to be edge
play. Other places consider

anything someone isn't completely familiar with doing on their own to be edge play and therefore needing extra supervision.

Edging

Foreplay that pushes someone to the edge of climax but denies them the ability to have an orgasm.

Egalitarian

A system where all parties are equal in power. In kink and/or polyamory relationship settings it is used to describe relationships where there may not be any D/s power exchange.

Electrosex / Electricity Play

Play that involves specific electricity related toys like a

_________________   ______________________

                    ____

_________________   ______________________

violet wand and TENS unit.

Emotional Triggers

Words, phrases, topics, or even sounds that can cause intense emotional responses.

Endorphins

A naturally occurring hormone in the human body that helps control and ease pain. In painful kink play this hormone can lessen that pain and create an opiate like high effect.

Enema

Use of liquid to help clear out the lower bowel often used to prepare for anal sex or play.

Energy Play

Form of play that focuses on using a person's own aura and energy to create and manipulate connection with another person.

E-Stim   Another term for TENS units
which send electrical signals
into the muscles to cause
contractions.

Etiquette   Common rules and guidelines
for engaging with fellow kinky
people in someone's local
community.

**Exclusive
Relationship**   A relationship that excludes
other people.

Exhibitionism   Fetish for being watched by
other people while engaging in
sex or kink activity.

**Extended
Family**   Refers to chosen family and
those who are connected but

not necessarily close the core person. For example, someone's best friend is chosen family but their best friend's sister may be extended family.

Eye Contact Restriction

Rules set up in power exchange relationships where the submissive partner is limited in the amount and type of eye contact they can make with other people.

Family

A group of people someone gets close to through relationships, friendships, play partners, and trusted community members.

Fear Play

Play that is centered around

fear and the adrenaline rush
that follows.

Feederism

Arousal from eating, feeding,
and gaining weight.

**FemDom /
Femme Domme**

A label used by some dominant
women to identify themselves:
Female Dominant - FemDom

Feminization

Play that involves dressing
someone in women's clothing
and feminine makeup to
encourage, or force, them to
be more feminine in scene.

Femme

Having the characteristics of
being feminine in appearance
and mannerisms.

Fetish

An object, activity, or situation

_________________   _________________

____

_________________   _________________

that causes sexual arousal.

Fetish Community

Community of people who are interested in fetish/kink/bdsm.

Fetlife

A popular social media website that calls itself the "social network for the bdsm, fetish, and kinky community."

Figging

Anal play that involves ginger root.

Fire Cupping

A form of cupping play that involves the use of fire to create the suction.

Fire Play

Play that involves small, controlled contacts with fire. The definition of "don't try this at home."

Fisting	Sexual play that involves putting a whole fist inside the vagina or anus.
Flagellation	Also known as flogging which involves impact play with floggers.
Flagging	Use of different colored handkerchiefs to signal what kind of sex or kinks someone is interested in, mainly used for finding new partners.
Flesh Hooks	Large piercing hooks that are used to pierce the skin for skin pulls and hook suspensions.
Floggers	Whip like impact toys that have multiple tails/falls similar to a cat o'nine tails, but with more falls. Materials vary from

a large range of leather to a wide selection of synthetics. While often confused for one, going into a dungeon and asking for a "whip" will get you a bullwhip, not a flogger. (See figure on pg 132)

Flogging

Also known as flagellation which involves impact play with floggers.

Flying

1. Term for when someone is suspended mid-air via bondage means.
2. Term used to describe the high-flying feeling that comes with subspace.

Foot Fetish / Worship

Play where someone's point of focus and source of arousal is someone else's feet.

**Forced
Orgasms**

Play that involves involuntary, forced orgasms that over time can become painful due to the constant contracting muscles.

Forniphilia

The fetish for being treated like human furniture, like a table or chair.

Funishment

Term used to describe "punishment" like impact play, or corporal punishment, that isn't actually being used to punish bad behavior but rather being treated like a game.

Furry

Someone who belongs to the Furry community, a group of people who identify with

_______________ _______________

____

_______________ _______________

anthropomorphic characters as
an extension of themselves.
Often seen wearing large
fur-suits of brightly colored
animals.

Gang Bang

Group sex of consecutive
rough intercourse of one
person on the receiving end
with multiple people as tops.

Gay

Someone who is sexually
attracted to people of the
same sex as themselves.

Gear

Umbrella term for kink
and fetish paraphernalia
from clothes to toys and
accessories.

**Gender
Identity**

How someone identifies in

_______________   _______________

____

_______________   _______________

____

terms of male vs female, both or neither, which previously was thought to be synonymous with biological sex. No longer the limited binary scale previously assumed, identity still has connections to societal gender roles and how someone fits within them.

Gender Play

Play that involves taking on gender roles, identity, and expression contrary to someone's base identity.

Genderqueer

Gender identity where someone is neither solely masculine or feminine, but may identify with both, neither, or parts of each.

Genitorture

Genital torture play, such as

cock and ball torture (CBT).

Gifted Leather   Leather clothing and accessories that are given as gifts as opposed to those that are "earned."

Girl   A title used mainly by submissive women in kink communities; counter to "Ma'am" which is for dominant women.

Glory Hole   Anonymous sexual encounters where someone puts their penis into a hole in a wall to receive manual stimulation or fellatio.

Golden Shower   The act of urinating on another person or being urinated on.

______________________   ______________________

____

______________________   ______________________

Gor/Gorean

A kink/bdsm lifestyle based on a series of science fiction books written by John Lange in 1966.

Gorean Slave Positions

Positions pulled from the "Gor" book series that are used by submissive/slave partners to show subservience. While "Gor" often receives credit for these positions, the origins date back much further. Salutes and attention stances are two examples of required body positionings between rulers, or high-ranking officials, and their subordinates.

Greysexual

Sexual identity on the asexual spectrum for someone who is not completely asexual but also does not experience sexual attraction the same way the average person does. The grey area between sexual attraction and no sexual attraction.

Group Sex — Sex involving more than 2 people, also known as an orgy.

Handler — Someone who manages the pets in pet play scenarios, like a dog handler in puppy play.

Hard Limits — A thing, phrase, or situation that is entirely off limits for someone; something that will never be consented to.

Heavy SM — Heavy sadomasochism; play that intends to involve a great deal of pain.

Hematolagnia To have a fetish for or to be aroused by blood.

Heteroromantic Someone who is romantically attracted to people of the "opposite" sex as themselves.

Heterosexual Someone who is sexually attracted to people of the "opposite" sex as themselves.

High Protocol A set of rules created by D/s couples that are used during formal occasions. This can include speech or eye contact restrictions, clothing limits, and more.

Hojojutsu Martial art involving the use of rope or cording to restrain someone. Originated in Japan.

Homoromantic	Someone who is romantically attracted to people of the same sex as themselves.
Homosexual	Someone who is sexually attracted to people of the same sex as themselves.
Hood	A mask that covers the whole head. Can be used for sensory deprivation, as fashion, or to alter one's image, like a pup hood.
Hook Suspension	Suspension done with use of multiple large hooks pierced into the skin.
Human Ashtray	Someone who enjoys either holding an ashtray or being the ashtray for ashes to be

_______________   _______________

____

_______________   _______________

dropped on their skin or even their tongue.

Humiliation

Engagement that breaks someone down at their core, affecting their self-worth.

Hypnosis

Play that involves induction and placing suggestions towards achieving an end kink goal, such as orgasm control via countdown.

Impact Play

A scene where someone hits (impacts) their partner with something, such as a paddle, flogger, crop, or bare hand (spanking).

Infantilism

Fetish where someone acts like an infant; in some cases, the participant may age-regress, in others it may be just role-play.

Interrogation Play

Use of interrogation techniques in a scene for the purpose of gaining information or a predetermined code word.

Intersex

Term used for anyone born with physical sexual characteristics that are atypical for the definitions of a male or female body.

Japanese Bondage

Style of bondage that originated in Japan, such as shibari, kinbaku, and hojojutsu.

Kajira

Originating from the "Gor" book series, female slave.

Kajirus Originating from the "Gor" book series, male slaves.

Kinbaku Having the literal definition of "tight binding." Term that is used to label a certain type of Japanese styled rope bondage.

Kink Activities of a sexual nature that fall outside of what is considered "normal" sexual behavior.

Kink Aware Phrase used to identify professionals who have a limited understanding of kink and BDSM.

Kink Friendly Professionals who are not just "kink aware" in having a limited understanding of kink, but more involved and able to have deeper conversations around kink as a whole.

Kinkster

Someone who is involved in the kink/BDSM lifestyle.

Kinky

To have kinks/fetishes.

Kitten

Someone who identifies as a cat or kitten in a pet play scenario.

Klismaphilia

Fetish for administering and/or receiving enemas.

Knife Play

Use of a knife or similar item that can replicate the feeling of a knife in play to create sensations that are sharp or scratchy. The purpose is typically not to actually cut the skin, which is a different type of play.

Lace
Delicate sheer fabric that is created through weaving fine threads such as silk and cotton.

Lactophilia
Fetish for breast milk.

Latex
Rubber sheeting used to create clothing that is known for being shiny and tight fitting.

Leather
1. Finished animal hides, such as cow, that is used to create clothing and kink gear from floggers and whips to harnesses and restraints, and more. 2. A subculture of kinky people who identify as "Leather," enjoy wearing leather, and at times claim to

be more involved in their local communities than the "average kinkster."

Leather Bar   A bar that is designed for and frequented by people who enjoy BDSM and leather.

Leatherman   A man who identifies as belonging to the Leather subculture.

Leatherperson   A person who identifies as belonging to the Leather subculture.

Leatherwoman   A woman who identifies as belonging to the Leather subculture.

Lesbian   A woman who is sexually attracted to other women.

Lifestyler   Someone who views kink and
fetishism as a lifestyle instead
of something engaged in every
once and a while.

Limits   Activities and encounters
that are outside of someone's
comfort zone.

Little   An adult who acts or role
plays as a child typically
aged from 1 to 12 years old.
This play is not related to
pedophilia.

Live In Slave   A submissive partner who lives
with their dominant partner in
a master and slave dynamic.

**Long Term
Relationship**   A relationship that is expected
to last for many years or has
no end date in sight.

__________________   __________________

          ____

__________________   __________________

          ____

Love Language	Ways that love is communicated from one person to another. The 5 love languages are: physical touch, words of affirmation, quality time, acts of service, and gifting.
Ma'am	An honorific often given to women or feminine presenting people as a sign of respect; shortened version of "madam."
Macrophilia	Fetish for role play including giant people, usually women, who are significantly larger than the other person.
Masc	A shortened version of the word "masculine."

_______________   ______________________

_______________   ______________________

____

Maschalagnia   Armpit fetishism; typically involves smelling and worship of them.

Masochism   To enjoy receiving pain. For some the enjoyment is sexual but it doesn't have to be.

Masochist   Someone who enjoys receiving pain.

Master   The dominant partner in a total power exchange master and slave relationships dynamic.

Master's Cover   A leather hat, originally created by Muir Cap Company, that is often used to designate dominance or mastery in formal leather uniforms.

_______________   _______________________

____

_______________   _______________________

____

| **Matriarchy** | Societal structure where women hold the majority of the authority and power positions, such as in government and other positions of privilege. |

| **Medical Play** | Play that involves medical equipment and/or roleplay. While sharps like needles and scalpels fall into this play type, they are not required. Play might also include things like uniforms, reflex hammers, restraints, and so on. |

| **Microphilia** | Fetish for role play including very small people or body parts. |

| **#MeToo** | Movement started in 2006 by Tarana Burke to end sexual |

harassment and abuses by lifting voices of survivors through solidarity and empathy.

Middle

An adult who acts or role plays as a teenage child typically aged from 13 to 17 years old. This play is not related to pedophilia.

Mind Fucks

A type of play that involves tricking the mind into believing that one thing is going to happen, only for something else to then happen instead. One of the best examples is in the "Punisher" movie where he convinces a guy that he's about to be burned only to instead touch him with a popsicle.

| **Mistress** | A title often given to women or femme presenting people. |

| **Mommy** | Title given to and used by people who might identify as a mother figure in Age Play or simply enjoy being called "Mommy." |

| **Monogamy** | A relationship type that contains only 2 people. |

| **Muir Cap** | A leather hat, originally created by Muir Cap Company, that is often used to designate dominance or mastery in formal leather uniforms. (See figure on pg 127) |

| **Mummification** | To mimic how mummies were wrapped as a form of play. Often this is accomplished with |

_______________   _____________________________

____

_______________   _____________________________

plastic wrap or cloth wraps covering the majority of the body.

Munch

A non-kink meeting for kinky people. Often held in a restaurant or bar as a way for people to meet in a non-play, less threatening setting. Due to the public nature of these meetings, fetish-wear is often discouraged.

Mutual Masturbation

Where two or more people masturbate while in close proximity of each other.

Needle Play

Play that involves needles temporarily being put in the skin, usually horizontally, for the sake of inflicting pain and/ or creating designs.

**Negative
Status**

When an STI panel (test)
comes back as negative. This
is alternative to saying "clean"
which puts a harsher, negative
connotation on those with
STI's.

Negotiation

A discussion had about an
upcoming scene so that all
parties involved are on the
same page with what will
happen during the scene. This
is the time to set boundaries
and discuss expectations.

New Guard

A term used for the "new
leather" crowd, often used for
younger groups of people in
contrast to "Old Guard."

Newbie

Someone who is brand new to

the kink/bdsm community.

Non-Monogamy   Relationships that do not stick to the rules of monogamy; this includes things like swinging, polyamory, cuckholds, and so on.

Nostril Strap   A strap that goes across the face, typically with hooks in the nose, that is meant to humiliate the wearer.

Novice   A beginner in the kink/bdsm world.

Nylons   Fetish for pantyhose, leggings, stockings, and similar accessories.

O-Ring   A circular, solid ring often used in collars or on jewelry to symbolize bdsm.

O-Ring Gag A gag that features an o-ring instead of a ball, leaving the mouth open and accessible.

Objectification A type of play that involves being treated like an object instead of a person.

Old Guard A term created to signify older leather people from where it was believed many protocols and traditions were derived.

Olfactophilia Arousal from various smells and scents.

Open Marriage A form of non-monogamy where two people are married and still have the ability to date and have relationships outside of their marriage.

Open Relationship

A form of non-monogamy where two people are in a relationship and still have the ability to date and have other relationships outside of their own.

Orgasm Control

Play that involves having control over someone's ability to orgasm both in denial of them and causing them.

Over The Knee

Play that occurs with the bottom being placed in the top's lap or "over the knee."

Ownership

Term used in dominant/ submissive relationships to lay claim to another person as property.

Paddle   A piece of equipment that
is usually made of wood or
another similar hard material
and shaped similar to a small
boat oar, though shapes and
designs do vary greatly. Used
in impact play or spanking
type scenes to hit the
bottom's butt.
(See figure on pg 132)

Pansexual   Someone has the capacity to
be attracted to all people,
where sex and gender are not
limiting factors.

Patriarchy   Societal structure where
men hold the majority of the
authority and power positions,
such as in government and

_______________   _______________________

                   ____

_______________   _______________________

other positions of privilege.

Pegging Play where a woman uses a strap-on to have anal sex with her partner.

Pet Play Role play where someone pretends to be an animal of their choosing through specialty gear and toys. This is not the same as being a furry.

Petition Paperwork used to request something from another person, such as petitioning for mentorship, ownership, training, and so on.

Phys-Dom A term used in online forums to describe a dominant who focuses on physical control more than psychological.

Piercing

Body modification that involves puncturing the skin and then inserting a metal hoop or stud jewelry that will remain in place.

Play

Activity between two or more people in a kink setting.

Play Partner

A relationship type that involves kink play but no romantic attachment or plans to become romantic.

Play Party

A setting or space where multiple people are getting together to play in one area. Can be held in private settings (like a house party) or in a more public setting (like an established dungeon).

__________   __________________

____

__________   __________________

Plushophilia	Fetish for stuffed animals.
Podophilia	Foot fetishism.
Polyam / Polyamory	Form of non-monogamy where partners are allowed to have multiple relationships.
Pony Play	Play that involves someone dressing up like a pony or horse. Some participate in pony shows that include agility competitions.
Pony Training	Training used to get a human pony ready for things like cart pulling or agility contests.
Position Training	Training used to teach a submissive partner various

positions for service such as how to sit, kneel, or present items.

Positive Status   When an STI panel (test) comes back as positive. This is alternative to saying "dirty" which puts a harsher, negative connotation on those with STI's.

Posture Collar   A collar that is designed to keep someone's head up and their neck straight, very similar to a c-collar in the medical field.
(See figure on pg 127-128)

Power Exchange   The term used to describe the authority exchange that happens in dominant/submissive relationships;

essentially who is in charge of what and how.

Predator/Prey   A dynamic that taps into someone's more primal nature as a hunter (predator) or prey. Some people revert to a specific animal, like a bear or wolf, some revert to primal human nature.

Predicament Bondage   Bondage that puts the bottom into a precarious situation where they must choose between two or more uncomfortable positions.

Pressure Points   Play that involves creating pain by applying pressure to tender spots on the body such as acupressure spots, nerve bundles, and overlapping muscles.

Professional Dominant Someone who is paid to act as a dominant for hire. They perform services like bossing someone around, topping for impact play, or any number of other play types.

Property Title given to someone who is "owned" by someone else in terms of a dominant/submissive, master/slave, or owner/property relationship.

Protocols A set of rules and expectations that are set to be done regularly in a dominant/submissive relationship.

__________   ________________

____

__________   ________________

____

Psych-Dom   A term used in online forums
to describe a dominant who
focuses on mental control
more than physical.

Pummeling   Impact play that revolves
around use of punches, kicks,
and similar hits from body
parts.

Punishment   Use of negative stimulus to
deter further misbehaving
after rules have been
broken. Often confused for
"funishment" which is light-
hearted rule breaking that is
met with play like a spanking.
Funishment is meant to be
enjoyed and fun, punishment is
not.

Puppy Play   Play that involves dressing

up and behaving like a dog or puppy.

Pup Hood

A hood designed to mimic a dog's face with ears and a snout/muzzle for humans participating in puppy play to feel and look more like the canine they're roleplaying as. (See figure on pg 128)

Pushing Limits

When someone (consensually) attempts to engage in activities that would normally fall under their soft or hard limit list in hopes to overcome their aversion.

Queening

Sexual act that involves a woman sitting and rubbing her genitals on the faces of a subservient partner.

| **Queer** | An umbrella term used to represent everyone in the LGBTQIA+ community. |

| **Questioning** | To be unsure of or undecided on a specific gender or sexual identity. |

| **Quirt** | An impact play toy that has a body similar to a short whip with two thick leather falls that come off the end. |

| **Reference** | An outside source of information used to learn more about a person, place, or thing. |

| **Relationship (Big R)** | Big R relationships are those that people think of when people are romantically involved together, like marriage. |

___________________   ___________________

                         ____

___________________   ___________________

(Little r)	Little r relationships are typically relationships that don't have a romantic component, like friendships or play partners.
Rhino Hide	When a masochist is able to take a lot of impact play giving the impression that they have "thick skin."
Rimming	Sexual activity that involves stimulating the outer ring of the anus.
Role Play	To pretend to be someone or something that you aren't normally.
Rubber	A material that is commonly used in kink toys as well as being made into clothing that

	can be restrictive and very shiny.
Rule #1	A common rule in many dominant/submissive relationships: "Take care of the property; the submissive is the most valuable property."
Rules	Restrictions and directions set in place in a dominant/submissive relationship that dictate how the relationship and all related matters will function.
Sadism	To enjoy inflicting pain on other people. For some causing pain involves a sexual component, but not always.
Sadist	Someone who enjoys inflicting

pain on other people.

**Sado-
masochism**

To enjoy inflicting pain on others as well as having pain inflicted on themselves. May or may not be connected to a sexual component.

Safe Call

A call set up before a date or get together that is designed to check on someone during the date.

Safe Signal

A non-verbal way of communicating that someone needs assistance during a scene.

Safer Sex

Formerly called "safe sex," safer sex is when extra steps are taken to reduce risk of STI's and pregnancy during

_______________ _______________________

____

_______________ _______________________

____

sex.

Safeword

A word or phrase used during a scene to stop or pause the activity when it has been negotiated that the bottom wants "no" or "stop" not to end the scene.

Scat

Play that involves fecal matter.

Scene

A kink play session.

Sensory Deprivation

Play that involves taking away senses like limiting sight with a blindfold, or limiting hearing with earplugs.

Sensual Play

Play that focuses on engaging the senses like using feathers

_______________   _______________

                    ____

_______________   _______________

                    ____

or varying temperatures on the skin.

Service   Acts of doing something to make the other person's life a little easier such as preparing meals, cleaning, and so on.

Service-Oriented   Someone whose main focus is providing acts of service for their partner.

Session   Another name for a scene. A time period of kink activity.

Sex Magick   Belief around the idea that sex can affect someone's energy and manifestation of such in the world.

Sex Work   Term used to replace

"prostitution" in describing those whose work involves sex.

Sexual Orientation   How someone identifies in their sexual attraction such as straight, gay, bisexual, etc.

Shaving   Use of a blade or razor to remove hair from the body.

Shoe Fetishism   Having a fetish for shoes as a whole or those of a particular style.

Signal Whip   A type of whip that has a cracker braided into the end of the thong rather than a fall.

Single Tail   Category of impact play toys that have a single fall, such as

_______________   _______________

____

_______________   _______________

a whip, rather than multiple falls, like a flogger.

Sir An honorific often given to men or masculine presenting people as a sign of respect.

Sissification Play that involves feminizing a man for the purpose of humiliation or degradation.

Slave The submissive partner in a total power exchange master and slave relationships dynamic.

Slave Contract A mock-up contract that is meant to simulate legally binding paperwork stating ownership between the dominant and submissive partners in a total power exchange relationship

Slave Training Time spent teaching the submissive partner in a total power exchange relationship about expectations in daily life and the relationship as a whole. Common training topics may include things like drink service, bedtime protocols, and so on.

Slavery In kink this is a consensual arrangement between adults to roleplay or act out the arrangement of one adult belonging completely to another.

Sling A piece of bondage equipment that resembles a hammock chair that is typically made

out of leather or rubber.
(See figure on pg 129)

Smart Ass Masochist

A phrase used to describe a person who uses sarcasm to encourage or invoke a response of funishment (feigned punishment).

Soft Limits

Activities that someone doesn't have much interest in but are not necessarily off the table completely.

Sounds

Thin, smooth metal rods that are used by inserting them into the urethra.

Spanking

Play that involves hitting someone on the butt with a bare hand.

**Spanking
Bench**   Dungeon furniture that is
                    designed to put the bottom
                    into a bent over position so
                    that the butt is exposed and
                    sticking out.

Spanking Skirt   A skirt with a hole cut out
                    in the back to expose the
                    wearer's butt.

Spanko   Someone's whose primary play
                    type is spankings.

**Speech
Restriction**   A set of rules within a
                    dominant and submissive
                    relationship where the
                    submissive is limited in who
                    they can talk to, what they
                    can say, or some other factor
                    related to their freedom to

_______________   _______________________

                   ____

_______________   _______________________

speak.

Spreader Bar A bar with cuffs on either end designed to separate the arms and/or legs from each other.

Squeak A latex fetishist. Named for the "squeaking" sound latex can make when it rubs against itself.

Squish A platonic, non-sexual crush. Term is often used by those in the Ace/Asexual spectrum.

St. Andrews Cross Dungeon furniture that is shaped like an X, commonly seen with tie points at the top and bottom to restrain the wrists and ankles.
(See figure on pg 129)

__________________   ______________________________

____

__________________   ______________________________

____

**Stand and
Model**   A phrase used to describe
                fetish events where there is
                little play involved and instead
                the focus is on dressing up in
                fetish-wear and mingling.

Stapling   Use of medical staples to
                inflict pain or bind someone.

Stigmatophilia A fetish for body modifications
                like piercings and tattoos.

Sting   Term used to describe one
                of the two major pain types.
                Sting is a pain sensation that
                feels sharp, often a surface
                level pain.

Stocks   Dungeon furniture designed to
                keep the head and both arms
                restrained, often in a standing

_______________   _____________________

                ____

_______________   _____________________

                ____

position.

Stoplight Safewords

A safeword system that operates with the use of red meaning stop, yellow meaning check-in, and green meaning go.

Straight

Heterosexual. Someone who is attracted to people on the opposite end of the binary gender scale.

Strap

An impact play item made from a length of leather, rubber, or similar flexible material; they often look very similar to a belt.

Strap-On

A dildo and harness combination designed to attach said dildo to the wearer's pelvis.

Submission   To hand over authority to
someone else.

Submissive   The person in a power
exchange relationship who
yields control to the other
partner(s).

Subspace   A state of being where a
natural high is achieved after
production of neurochemicals
like endorphins and adrenaline
in a kink scene.

Surrender   To give up or yield.

Suspension   Use of rope or other binding
methods to hang someone
mid-air.

Suspension

_____________   _____________

     ____

_____________   _____________

Cuffs	Bondage cuffs that are used to hang/suspend someone from the wrists or ankles. (See figure on pg 128)
Sutures	Medical equipment used to close wounds via string and needles. In kink setting they can be used for decorating the skin or binding.
Swinging	A form of ethical non-monogamy where the focus is additional sexual partners rather than romantic involvement.
Switch	Someone who likes to top and bottom, or someone who identifies as both dominant and submissive.

Tawse

An impact play item that resembles a paddle, typically made of leather, with a split or forked end.
(See figure on pg 133)

TENS Unit

Transcutaneous electrical nerve stimulation unit. A piece of medical equipment that operates by sending electrical pulses through the skin and muscles of the wearer, designed for pain relief.

Teratophilia

Fetish for or attraction to monsters, sometimes meaning monstrous people, other times meaning literal monsters like vampires, wolf man, Frankenstein's monster, etc.

Thong

The main body of a single-tail

whip.

Thud

Term used to describe one of the two major pain types. Thud is a pain sensation that feels dull, often a deeper, under the surface of the skin level pain.

Top

To be on the giving end of an activity; topping is not the same as dominating. For example: to top for flogging means you are flogging the other person.

Topping From The Bottom

A phrase used to describe when a bottom was being too demanding mid-scene. Over time the phrase is being phased out in exchange for encouraging more communication during play.

Topspace

A state of being where a natural high is achieved after production of neurochemicals like endorphins and adrenaline in a kink scene.

Torture

S&M play that is intended to be particularly painful and hard to push through.

Toys

Umbrella term used for kink gear.

Trainee

Someone who has taken on the role of learning kink/bdsm from another person.

Training

Process by which someone learns kink/bdsm from

another person either as a
peer mentorship or teaching
a submissive their role in
a dominant and submissive
relationship.

Transgender   Someone who identifies as a
gender other than the one
they were assigned at birth.

Triad   A polyamorous relationship
with three people.

Trichophilia   Fetish for hair.

Two Spirit   A third gender option that is
rooted in indigenous, native
American people.

Uniforms   Assignment of specific clothing
to be worn during scenes or
whenever suits those involved

_____________   ___________________

____

_____________   ___________________

____

in the relationship.

Urethral Sound Thin, smooth metal rods that are used by inserting them into the urethra.

Urolagnia Also known as "watersports." Someone who enjoys being urinated on or urinating on others.

Vampire Glove Gloves that have sharp, pointed spikes in the fingertips that deliver a light scratching sensation up to the ability to puncture the skin.

Vanilla Non-kinky. Someone who isn't involved in the kink lifestyle or community.

Verbal Abuse To attack or manipulate

_______________   _______________

____

_______________   _______________

someone using words in such
a manner that it causes
detriment to the other person.

**Verbal
Humiliation**

Engagement that breaks
someone down at their core,
affecting their self-worth
through words.

Vested

The achievement of earning
your leather vest in social
circles involved with the
Leather lifestyle.

Violet Wand

A piece of equipment that
produces low amperage
electrical shock that feels
similar to constant static
shock for the purpose
of sensual and/or sexual
satisfaction.

____

____

____

**Vore /
Vorarephilia**   Arousal to the thought or
                   idea of being eaten or eating
                   someone whole.

Voyeurism   Fetish for watching other
                   people engage in sex or kink
                   activity.

**Wartenburg Wheel /
Pinwheel**   A piece of medical equipment
                   that resembles a pinwheel with
                   small spikes sticking out from
                   a central spoke that is used to
                   check nerve ending response.

Waterboarding A form of torture that involves
                   covering the person's face and
                   pouring water over it to cause
                   the person to feel like they're
                   drowning.

______________   ________________________

                   ____

______________   ________________________

Watersports   Play that involves someone urinating on the other person.

Wax   Moldable, meltable substance used for temperature or sensation play. The safest waxes for kink play are soy and paraffin because of their low melting point.

Wax Play   Play that involves pouring or dripping melted wax over the body.

Weekend Warrior   Term used to describe people who engage in kink play on occasion or part time rather than it being a regular part of their lives. Someone who goes to their local dungeon or kink event as a break from daily life.

Weights   Any weighted material that
                     can be used to add or apply
                     external mass in a kink scene.

Whipping   Any kink scene that involves
                     whip-like impact play
                     implements.

Whips   Shortened term for single-tail
                     whips.

Worship   To express admiration or
                     reverence for someone.

Wrapping   When a flexible impact play
                     toy, like a whip or flogger,
                     wraps around the side of the
                     body or passes by the intended
                     target area. For example, when
                     a hit that was meant to strike

___________________ ___________________________

                     ____

___________________ ___________________________

                     ____

the butt wraps around and hits
the hip instead.

**Your Kink Is Not
My Kink**

A phrase used to lessen
the stigma involved when
discussing kinks and fetishes
that do not align with your
own.

Zentai Suit

A skin-tight suit that covers
the entire body, including the
head, hands, and feet.

Hanky Code

What is hanky code?

"Hanky code" is a non-verbal method of communicating interests and desires through visual cues using different colored handkerchiefs stuck in the back pocket of the person looking for play. Each color has it's own meaning as well as which pocket the handkerchief is in. The left pocket typically signals a top with the right signalling a bottom for said activity.

Red   **Left:** Fisting top
       Right: Fisting bottom

Maroon: **Left:** Top for cutting play
       Right: Bottom for cutting play

Orange   **Left:** Anything, anytime, anywhere
(not anyone)
       Right: Nothing right now

Yellow   **Left:** Watersports top
       Right: Watersports bottom, looking to be peed on

Green   **Left:** Sex worker, available for hire
       Right: "John" looking to hire

Hunter Green

Left: Daddy
Right: Looking for a daddy

Teal

Left: CBT top
Right: CBT bottom

Blue

Left: Cop
Right: Badge bunny, looking for a cop

Light Blue

Left: Looking for oral sex
Right: Looking to perform oral sex

Purple

Left: Needle play top
Right: Needle play bottom

Fuschia

Left: Spanking top
Right: Spanking bottom

Light Pink

Left: Dildo top
Right: Didlo bottom

Dark Pink

Left: Breast/tit torture top
Right: Breast/tit torture bottom

Black

Left: Heavy S&M top, causes pain

Right: Heavy S&M bottom,
likes receiving pain

Grey   **Left:** Bondage top
Right: Bondage bottom

Brown   **Left:** Scat play top
Right: Scat play bottom

Gold   **Left:** Couple looking for third
Right: Single looking for couple

Silver Lame   **Left:** Celebrity chaser
Right: Celebrity

What else is out there?
This list contains some of the most commonly
used hanky code signals, not all of them. There
are always new signals being added and new ways
to represent your interests. Add yours below.

_______________   _________________________

                   ____

_______________   _________________________

Reference Images & Illustrations

Wearables & Bondage Gear

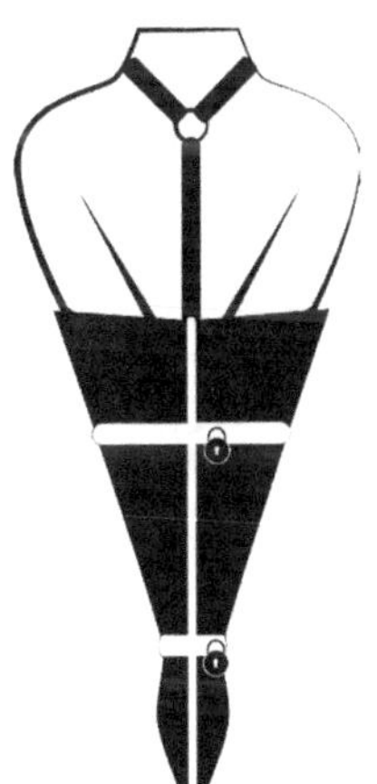

Armbinder - Info on
pg 21

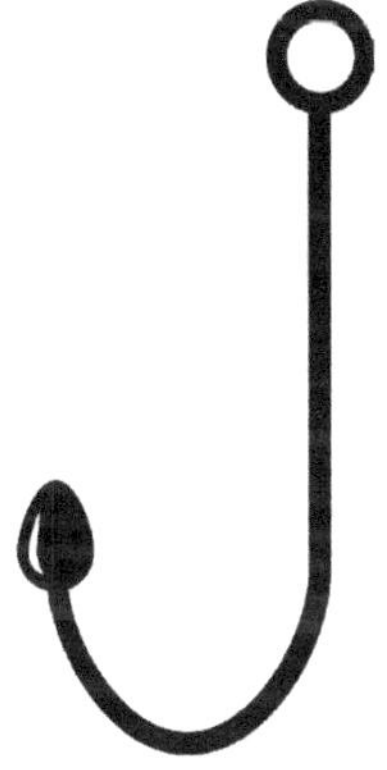

Anal Hook - Info on
pg 20

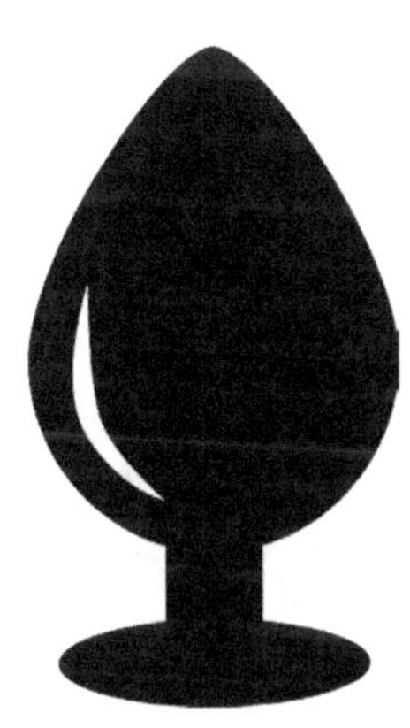

Butt Plug - Info on
pg 30

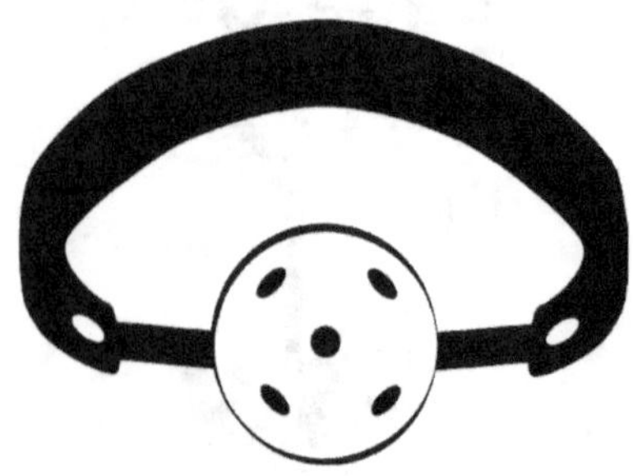

Ball Gag - Info on pg 23

Bllindfold - Info on
pg 24-25

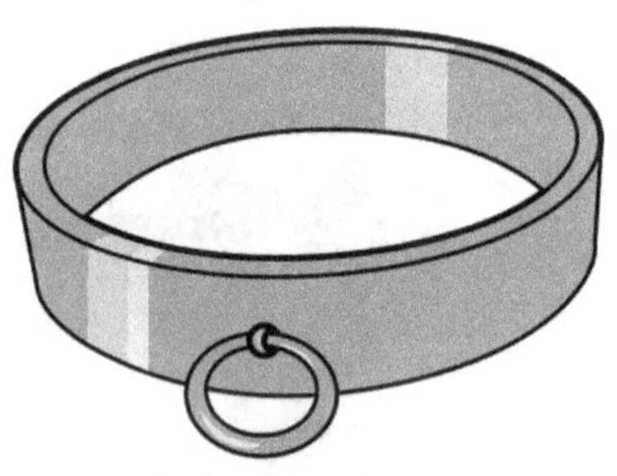

Collar - Info on pg 35

Chastity Cage - Info on
pg 33

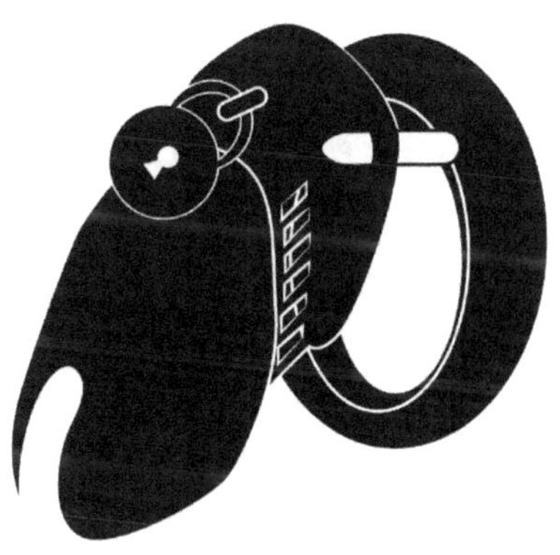

Muir Cap - Info on
pg 73

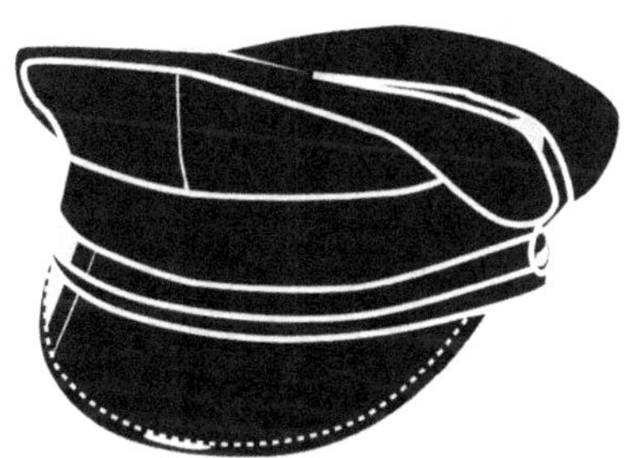

Posture Collar (decora-
tive) - Info on pg 83

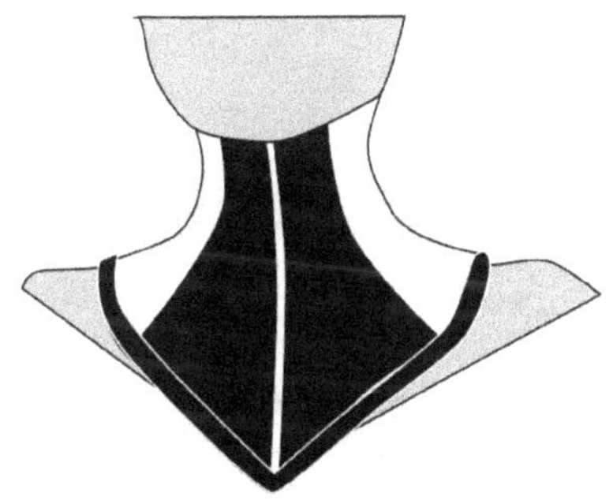

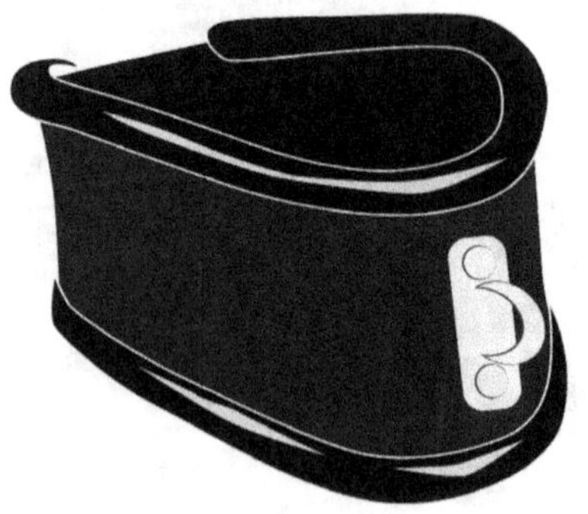

Posture Collar (struc-
tural) - Info on pg 84

Puppy Hood - Info on
pg 87

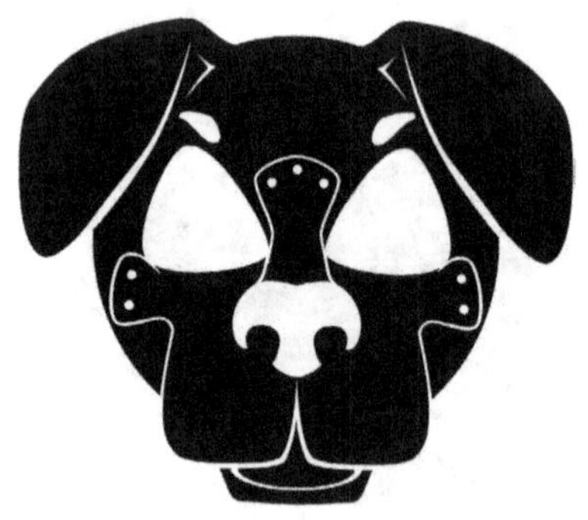

Suspension Cuff - Info
on pg 103

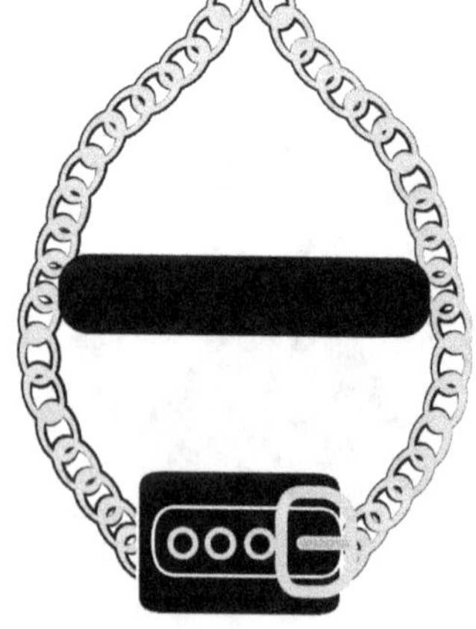

Dungeon Furniture

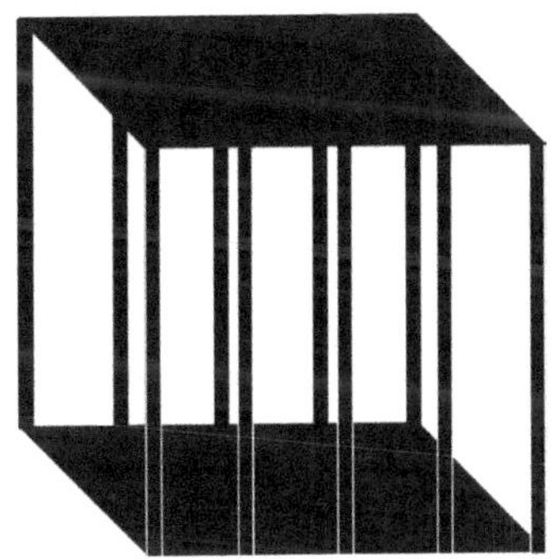

Cage - Info on pg 30

Sling - Info on pg 96

St. Andrew's Cross -
Info on pg 99

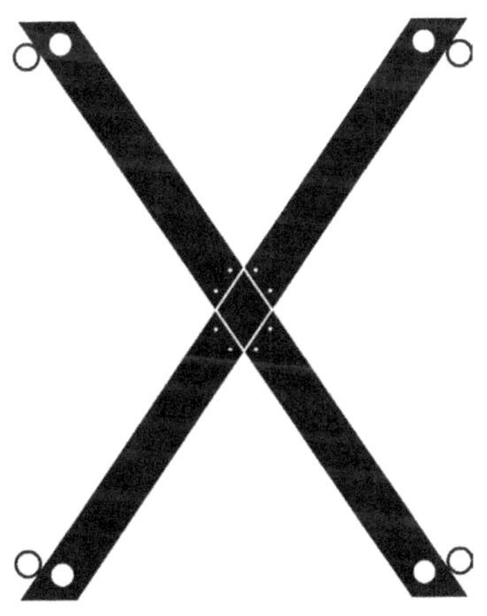

Impact Play & SM Gear

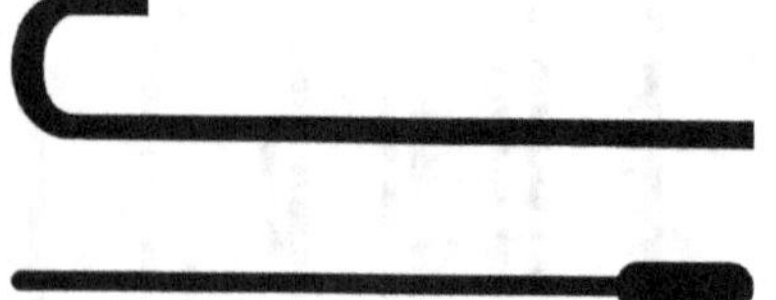

Canes - Info on
pg 30-31

Cat O'Nine Tails -
Info on pg 32-33

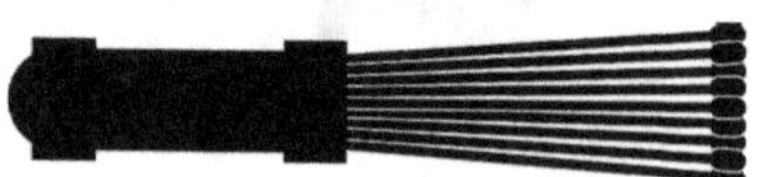

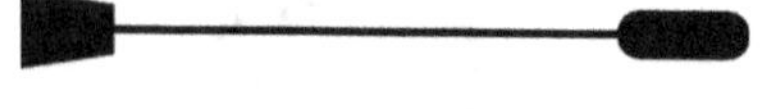

Crop - Info on pg 39-40

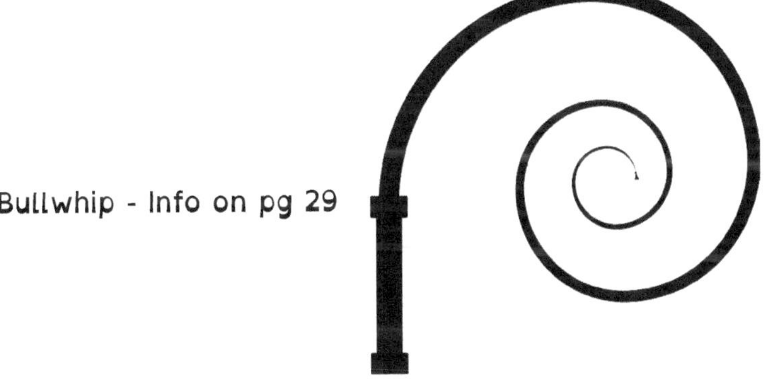

Bullwhip - Info on pg 29

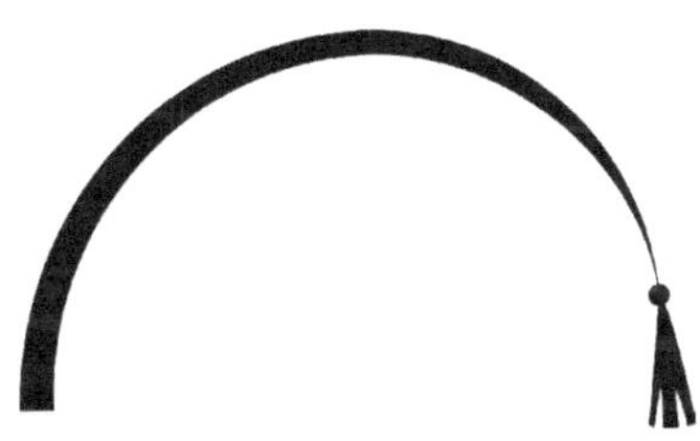

Cracker - Info on pg 39

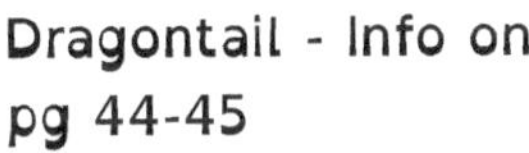

Dragontail - Info on
pg 44-45

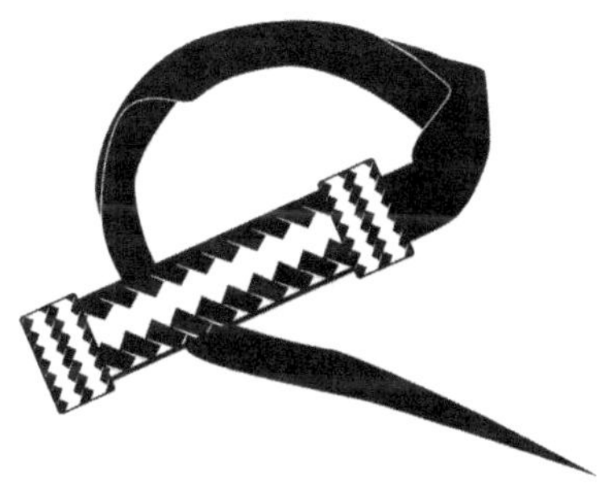

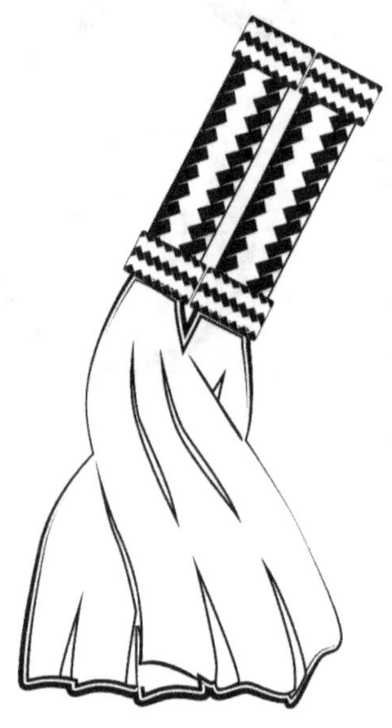

Flogger - Info on pg 53

Paddle - Info on pg 79

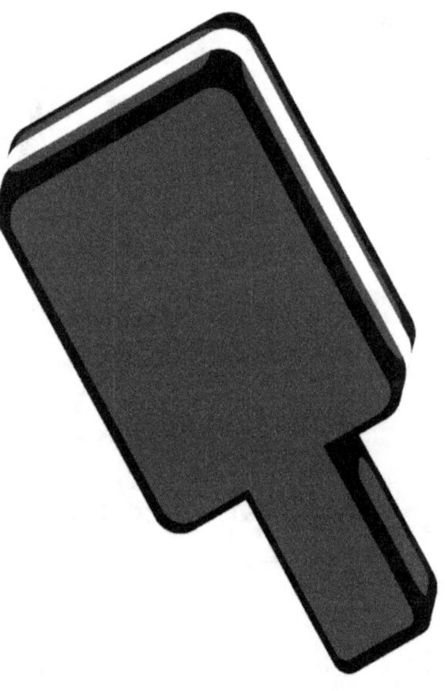

Clothespins - Info on
pg 34

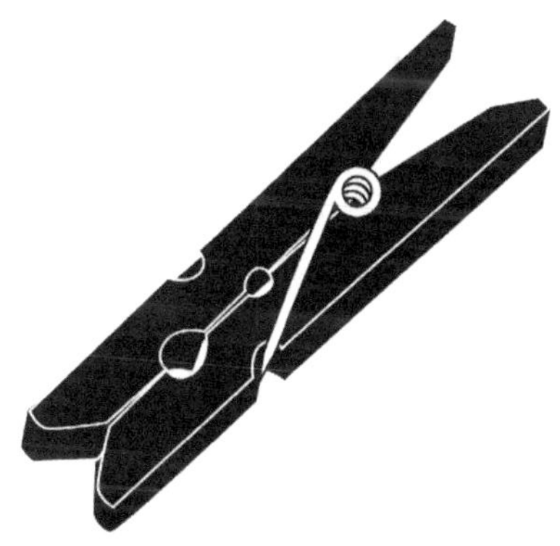

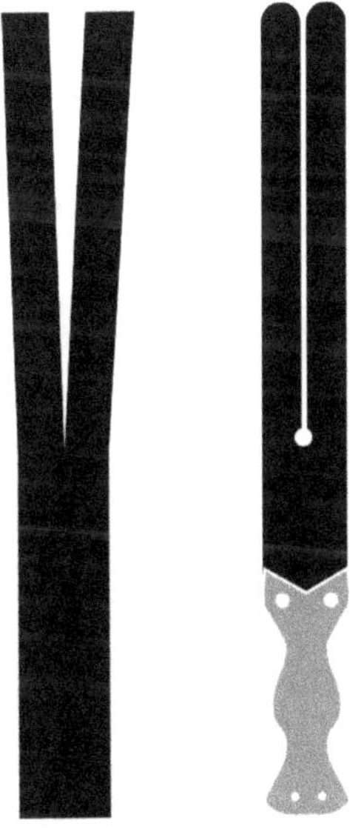

Tawse - Info on
pg 104

Use the following pages to add images of your favorite kink gear or related topics. Draw, cut and paste photos, or find other creative methods to display them.

About the
Author

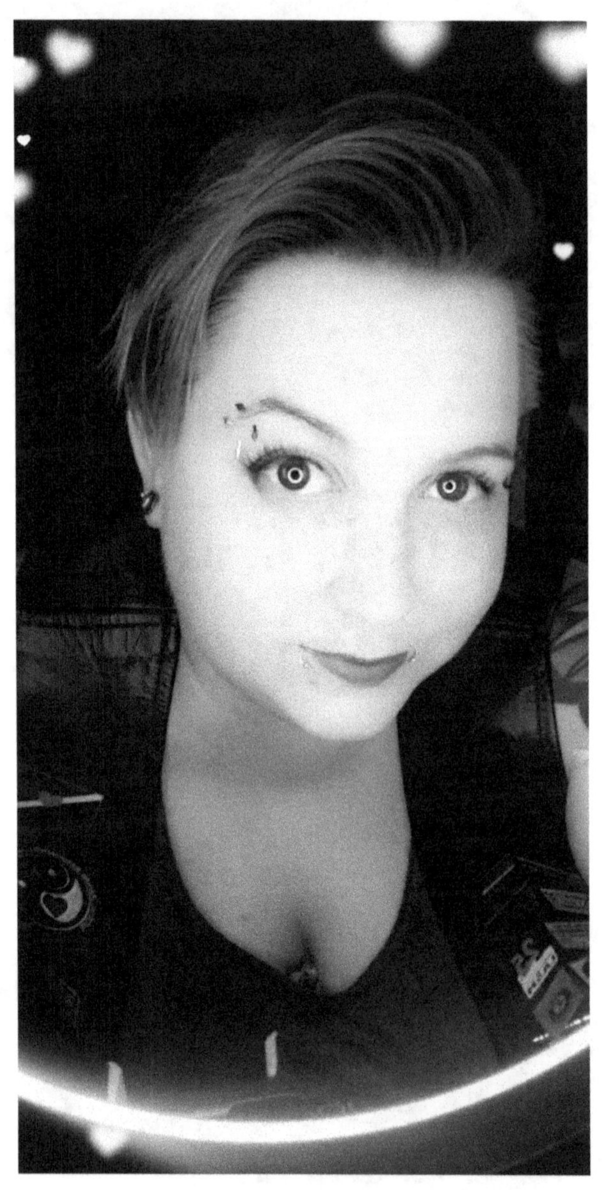

Ignixia is an internationally renowned professional kink educator and leather-woman who was the owner and sole-operator of an award-winning leather business designed around creating custom, quality leather goods that are affordable to all. She has used her skills as a leatherworker to create the Kinkability toy line, first of its kind fetish gear designed for those with disabilities. As someone who lives with chronic pain, along with her partner, she uses her experiences to help others with chronic pain through an online support group and classes designed to make daily life and kink easier to manage.

While leatherwork had provided a means to live, education and outreach fuel her passion for life. In one 5 year span she shared that passion by teaching at over 50 major kink conferences. When not traveling to teach at kink conventions, she volunteers 2 days per week at the Woodshed Orlando as a DM and educator. Locally she has also been a founding member and Co-Chair of NLA-Orlando, Co-Founder of WiLO (Women in Leather Orlando), Co-Creator of CFL Littles, and a supporter of WinK (Women in Kink), Dominant's Roundtable, and multiple under 35 groups.

In addition to donating products to multiple events' charity funds, she is the creator of over 100 kink/fetish based clothing designs including #KinkyCoexist and dozens of "Pride" Facebook profile frames used by thousands around the world. One of her latest endeavors has been the creation and management of Kink Positive, a project designed to promote kink and sex positive thinking through education by joining efforts with other educators, vendors, and events to maximize reach. Most recently it was even rumored that she put together a book!

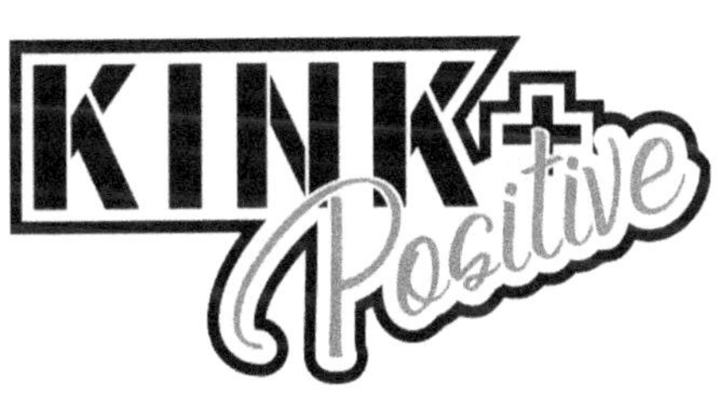